101 HOMEMADE BEAUTY RECIPES

From Pantry to Potion: DIY Beauty Elixirs

Melody Satin

INTRODUCTION

In today's world, where the beauty industry is saturated with products claiming miraculous results, it's easy to get lost in the myriad of choices. However, amidst the glittering aisles of commercial products, there's a rising trend that's taking us back to our roots: homemade beauty products. This movement isn't just about nostalgia or a return to simpler times; it's about understanding what goes onto our skin, the largest organ of our body, and ensuring that it's as natural and toxin-free as possible.

◆ ◆ ◆

The Benefits of Homemade Beauty Products

1. Transparency of Ingredients: One of the most significant advantages of homemade beauty products is knowing exactly what's in them. There's no deciphering of complex chemical names or wondering about potential side effects.

2. Cost-Effective: Often, making products at home can be more economical in the long run. Investing in a few quality ingredients can yield multiple batches of your favorite beauty product.

3. Customization: Everyone's skin is unique. Homemade products allow for personalization based on individual needs, be it for sensitive skin, specific skin issues, or personal scent preferences.

4. Eco-Friendly: By making products at home, you can reduce the environmental impact of packaging and the carbon footprint associated with transporting goods.

5. Freshness: Just like fresh food is often more nutritious, freshly made beauty products can offer more potent benefits since there's no long shelf life or need for preservatives.

6. Empowerment: There's a certain empowerment in taking control of your beauty regimen, understanding the science behind it, and being self-reliant.

◆ ◆ ◆

Safety Precautions and Best Practices

1. Patch Test: Before applying any homemade product all over your face or body, always do a patch test on a small area of skin to check for any allergic reactions.

2. Preservation: While homemade products don't contain commercial preservatives, it's essential to ensure they don't become breeding grounds for bacteria. Always use clean hands and tools, and consider natural preservatives like rosemary antioxidant extract or vitamin E.

3. Storage: Store products in a cool, dry place. Refrigeration can extend the shelf life of many homemade beauty products.

4. Research: Before diving into DIY beauty, research the ingredients you plan to use. Some natural ingredients can still be potent or irritating to some skin types.

5. Avoid Contamination: Always use sterilized containers for storing your products. Avoid dipping wet fingers into products to prevent mold and bacterial growth.

6. Expiration: Remember, without commercial preservatives, homemade products have a shorter shelf life. Use them promptly and be aware of any changes in smell, texture, or color.

7. Educate Yourself: While essential oils offer many benefits, they can be potent. Educate yourself about dilution rates and potential skin sensitivities.

◆ ◆ ◆

Embracing homemade beauty products is not just a trend; it's a lifestyle choice that prioritizes health, well-being, and a deeper connection to the ingredients we use. As with anything, knowledge is power, so equip yourself with the right information and enjoy the journey back to nature's lap.

CHAPTER 1: FACIAL CARE

Facial care is the cornerstone of any beauty regimen. The face is our most visible feature, and it's exposed to environmental factors daily. Using natural ingredients can help nourish the skin, ensuring it remains healthy, vibrant, and youthful. This chapter will guide you through a series of homemade recipes tailored for facial care, from cleansers to masks.

◆ ◆ ◆

1.1 Gentle Oatmeal Cleanser

Ingredients:

- 1/2 cup ground oatmeal

- 1/4 cup milk or water

- 1 tbsp honey

Instructions:

1. Mix the ground oatmeal and honey in a bowl.

2. Slowly add milk or water until a paste forms.

3. Apply to the face in circular motions, avoiding the eyes.

4. Rinse with warm water and pat dry.

Benefits: Oatmeal is known for its soothing properties, making it perfect for sensitive skin. Honey acts as a natural moisturizer and has antibacterial properties.

1.2 Honey and Lemon Brightening Mask

Ingredients:

- 2 tbsp raw honey

- 1 tbsp fresh lemon juice

Instructions:

1. In a bowl, combine honey and lemon juice.

2. Apply the mixture to a clean face, avoiding the eye area.

3. Leave on for 15-20 minutes.

4. Rinse off with warm water.

Benefits: Lemon juice acts as a natural exfoliant and brightener, while honey moisturizes and soothes the skin.

1.3 Green Tea Toner

Ingredients:

- 1 green tea bag

- 1 cup boiling water

- 1 tbsp witch hazel (optional)

Instructions:

1. Steep the green tea bag in boiling water for 5 minutes.

2. Remove the tea bag and allow the tea to cool.

3. Add witch hazel if desired.

4. Transfer to a clean bottle. Use a cotton pad to apply to the face after cleansing.

Benefits: Green tea is rich in antioxidants that can help reduce skin inflammation and redness. Witch hazel acts as an astringent, tightening the skin and pores.

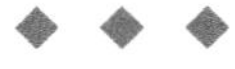

1.4 Avocado Moisturizing Mask

Ingredients:

- 1/2 ripe avocado

- 1 tbsp yogurt

- 1 tsp olive oil

Instructions:

1. Mash the avocado in a bowl.

2. Mix in yogurt and olive oil until smooth.

3. Apply to the face, avoiding the eyes.

4. Leave on for 20 minutes, then rinse with warm water.

Benefits: Avocado is rich in healthy fats and vitamins that nourish the skin. Yogurt contains lactic acid, which can exfoliate and smooth the skin, while olive oil moisturizes.

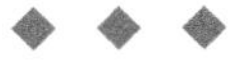

1.5 Coffee Grounds Exfoliating Scrub

Ingredients:

- 2 tbsp used coffee grounds

- 1 tbsp coconut oil

- 1 tsp brown sugar

Instructions:

1. Mix all ingredients in a bowl.

2. Gently massage onto the face in circular motions.

3. Rinse with warm water.

Benefits: Coffee grounds and brown sugar act as natural exfoliants, while coconut oil moisturizes.

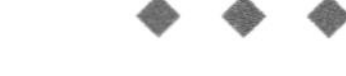

1.6 Cucumber Hydrating Mask

Ingredients:

- 1/2 cucumber, pureed
- 2 tbsp aloe vera gel

Instructions:

1. Blend cucumber until smooth.

2. Mix with aloe vera gel.

3. Apply to face and leave on for 20 minutes.

4. Rinse with cool water.

Benefits: Cucumber and aloe vera both have hydrating and soothing properties, perfect for dry or irritated skin.

1.7 Rosewater Setting Spray

Ingredients:

- 1/2 cup rosewater

- 1/4 cup distilled water

- 1 tsp glycerin

Instructions:

1. Combine all ingredients in a spray bottle.

2. Shake well before each use.

3. Spritz onto face after makeup application.

Benefits: Rosewater refreshes and hydrates the skin, while glycerin helps set makeup.

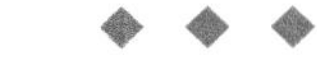

1.8 Charcoal Detoxifying Mask

Ingredients:

- 1 tsp activated charcoal powder

- 1 tsp bentonite clay

- 2 tbsp water or apple cider vinegar

Instructions:

1. Mix charcoal and clay in a bowl.

2. Slowly add water or apple cider vinegar to form a paste.

3. Apply to face, avoiding eyes.

4. Leave on for 10 minutes and rinse.

Benefits: Activated charcoal draws out impurities, and bentonite clay helps detoxify the skin.

1.9 Almond and Honey Cleanser

Ingredients:

- 2 tbsp ground almonds

- 1 tbsp honey

- 1 tsp milk

Instructions:

1. Mix all ingredients to form a paste.

2. Apply to face in circular motions.

3. Rinse with warm water.

Benefits: Almonds gently exfoliate, honey moisturizes, and milk soothes the skin.

❖ ❖ ❖

1.10 Chamomile Soothing Face Mist

Ingredients:

- 1 chamomile tea bag

- 1 cup boiling water

- 1 tsp glycerin

Instructions:

1. Steep chamomile tea in boiling water for 5 minutes.

2. Allow to cool and add glycerin.

3. Transfer to a spray bottle.

4. Mist face whenever you need a refresh.

Benefits: Chamomile has calming properties, making it perfect for reducing redness and irritation.

With these 10 recipes, you have a comprehensive facial care regimen using natural ingredients. Each recipe can be tailored to specific skin types or concerns, and you can experiment with different ingredients to find what works best for your skin.

CHAPTER 2: HAIR CARE

Hair is often referred to as one's crowning glory. It's not just about aesthetics; healthy hair is a reflection of good health and proper care. This chapter delves into homemade recipes that cater to various hair types and concerns, ensuring your locks remain lustrous and strong.

◆ ◆ ◆

2.1 Coconut Oil Deep Conditioner

Ingredients:

- 3 tbsp coconut oil

- 1 tbsp honey

- 1 tbsp aloe vera gel

Instructions:

1. Warm coconut oil slightly until it's liquid.

2. Mix in honey and aloe vera gel.

3. Apply to damp hair, focusing on the ends.

4. Leave on for 30 minutes, then shampoo out.

Benefits: Coconut oil penetrates hair shafts, providing deep moisture. Honey adds shine, and aloe vera soothes the scalp.

◆ ◆ ◆

2.2 Apple Cider Vinegar Hair Rinse

Ingredients:

- 2 tbsp apple cider vinegar

- 1 cup water

Instructions:

1. Mix apple cider vinegar with water.

2. After shampooing, pour the mixture over your hair.

3. Rinse thoroughly.

Benefits: Apple cider vinegar balances the scalp's pH and clarifies hair, removing product buildup.

◆ ◆ ◆

2.3 Herbal Hair Growth Serum

Ingredients:

- 2 tbsp castor oil

- 5 drops rosemary essential oil

- 5 drops lavender essential oil

Instructions:

1. Mix all ingredients in a small bottle.

2. Apply a few drops to the scalp and massage gently.

3. Leave overnight or wash out after an hour.

Benefits: Castor oil promotes hair growth, while rosemary and lavender stimulate the scalp and improve circulation.

$$\blacklozenge \quad \blacklozenge \quad \blacklozenge$$

2.4 Banana Hair Mask for Frizzy Hair

Ingredients:

- 1 ripe banana

- 2 tbsp yogurt

- 1 tbsp honey

Instructions:

1. Mash the banana and mix with yogurt and honey.

2. Apply to hair, covering from roots to tips.

3. Leave on for 30 minutes, then rinse and shampoo.

Benefits: Banana moisturizes and smoothens hair, yogurt adds shine, and honey acts as a humectant.

$$\blacklozenge \quad \blacklozenge \quad \blacklozenge$$

2.5 Chamomile Brightening Rinse for Blondes

Ingredients:

- 2 chamomile tea bags

- 2 cups boiling water

Instructions:

1. Steep chamomile tea bags in boiling water.

2. Allow to cool.

3. After shampooing, rinse hair with the chamomile infusion.

4. Do not rinse out; let hair dry naturally.

Benefits: Chamomile naturally brightens blonde hair and adds shine.

2.6 Avocado and Egg Hair Treatment

Ingredients:

- 1 ripe avocado

- 1 egg yolk

Instructions:

1. Mash avocado and mix with the egg yolk.

2. Apply to damp hair.

3. Leave on for 20 minutes, then rinse and shampoo.

Benefits: Avocado nourishes hair with vitamins and fats, while egg yolk adds protein, strengthening hair strands.

2.7 Rosemary Scalp Treatment for Dandruff

Ingredients:

- 2 tbsp olive oil

- 5 drops rosemary essential oil

Instructions:

1. Warm olive oil slightly and mix with rosemary oil.

2. Apply to the scalp and massage.

3. Leave on for 30 minutes, then shampoo.

Benefits: Rosemary has antifungal properties, and olive oil moisturizes the scalp, reducing flakes.

2.8 Flaxseed Hair Gel

Ingredients:

- 2 tbsp flaxseeds

- 1 cup water

Instructions:

1. Boil flaxseeds in water until a gel-like consistency forms.

2. Strain and let cool.

3. Apply to hair as a natural styling gel.

Benefits: Flaxseed gel provides a natural hold without drying out the hair.

◆ ◆ ◆

2.9 Aloe Vera Scalp Soother

Ingredients:

- 2 tbsp aloe vera gel

- 5 drops peppermint essential oil

Instructions:

1. Mix aloe vera gel with peppermint oil.

2. Apply to the scalp for a cooling sensation.

3. Rinse after 15 minutes or leave in.

Benefits: Aloe vera hydrates and soothes the scalp, while peppermint provides a refreshing feel.

◆ ◆ ◆

2.10 Beer Hair Rinse for Volume

Ingredients:

- 1/2 cup flat beer

- 1 cup water

Instructions:

1. Mix beer with water.

2. After shampooing, pour the mixture over your hair.

3. Rinse thoroughly.

Benefits: Beer contains proteins that can add volume and shine to limp hair.

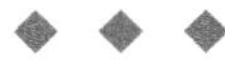

Your hair deserves as much care and attention as any other part of your body. With these natural recipes, you can address various hair concerns without the use of harsh chemicals. Remember to always do a patch test when trying out new ingredients to ensure no allergic reactions. Embrace the beauty of natural hair care and enjoy the benefits it brings!

CHAPTER 3: BODY CARE

The skin is the body's largest organ, and while facial care often takes the spotlight, the rest of the body deserves equal attention. This chapter focuses on nourishing and pampering the skin from the neck down, ensuring it remains soft, hydrated, and radiant.

◆ ◆ ◆

3.1 Lavender Bath Salts

Ingredients:

- 1 cup Epsom salt

- 1/2 cup sea salt

- 10 drops lavender essential oil

- A few dried lavender buds (optional)

Instructions:

1. Mix salts in a bowl.

2. Add lavender essential oil and mix well.

3. Sprinkle in dried lavender buds if desired.

4. Store in an airtight container. Add a handful to a warm bath and relax.

Benefits: Epsom salt helps soothe muscles, sea salt detoxifies, and lavender promotes relaxation.

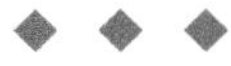

3.2 Almond Oil Body Lotion

Ingredients:

- 1/2 cup almond oil

- 1/4 cup coconut oil

- 1/4 cup beeswax

- 10 drops of your favorite essential oil (e.g., rose, jasmine)

Instructions:

1. In a double boiler, melt beeswax and oils together.

2. Remove from heat and let cool slightly.

3. Add essential oil and whisk until smooth.

4. Pour into a jar and let set.

Benefits: Almond and coconut oils moisturize deeply, while beeswax locks in hydration.

3.3 Brown Sugar Body Scrub

Ingredients:

- 1 cup brown sugar

- 1/2 cup olive oil or coconut oil

- 5 drops vanilla essential oil (optional)

Instructions:

1. Mix all ingredients in a bowl.

2. Store in an airtight container.

3. Use in the shower, scrubbing in circular motions and rinse.

Benefits: Brown sugar exfoliates dead skin cells, and the oils moisturize.

◆ ◆ ◆

3.4 Rose Water Body Mist

Ingredients:

- 1 cup rose water

- 1/4 cup witch hazel

- 10 drops rose essential oil

Instructions:

1. Combine all ingredients in a spray bottle.

2. Shake well before each use.

3. Mist over body for a refreshing scent.

Benefits: Rose water and rose essential oil soothe and hydrate skin, while witch hazel tones.

◆ ◆ ◆

3.5 Shea Butter Hand Cream

Ingredients:

- 1/2 cup shea butter

- 1/4 cup coconut oil

- 1/4 cup almond oil

- 10 drops lavender essential oil

Instructions:

1. In a double boiler, melt shea butter and oils.

2. Remove from heat and let cool slightly.

3. Add lavender essential oil and mix.

4. Pour into a jar and let set.

Benefits: Shea butter deeply moisturizes, and the oils nourish the skin. Lavender adds a calming scent.

3.6 Eucalyptus Foot Soak

Ingredients:

- 1 cup Epsom salt

- 1/2 cup baking soda

- 10 drops eucalyptus essential oil

Instructions:

1. Mix all ingredients in a bowl.

2. Add to a basin of warm water.

3. Soak feet for 15-20 minutes.

Benefits: Epsom salt relaxes tired feet, baking soda softens, and eucalyptus refreshes.

3.7 Coffee Cellulite Scrub

Ingredients:

- 1 cup coffee grounds

- 1/2 cup sugar

- 1/2 cup coconut oil

Instructions:

1. Mix all ingredients to form a paste.

2. In the shower, scrub areas with cellulite in circular motions.

3. Rinse off.

Benefits: Coffee stimulates circulation, sugar exfoliates, and coconut oil moisturizes.

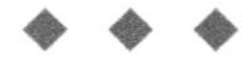

3.8 Calendula Healing Salve

Ingredients:

- 1/2 cup calendula-infused oil

- 1/4 cup beeswax

- 10 drops lavender essential oil

Instructions:

1. In a double boiler, melt beeswax into calendula oil.

2. Remove from heat and add lavender oil.

3. Pour into small tins or jars and let set.

Benefits: Calendula promotes skin healing, beeswax protects, and lavender soothes.

3.9 Aloe Vera Sunburn Gel

Ingredients:

- 1 cup aloe vera gel

- 5 drops peppermint essential oil

- 5 drops lavender essential oil

Instructions:

1. Mix all ingredients in a bowl.

2. Store in a cool place.

3. Apply to sunburned areas for relief.

Benefits: Aloe vera cools and heals, while peppermint and lavender soothe burned skin.

◆ ◆ ◆

3.10 Chamomile Body Oil

Ingredients:

- 1 cup jojoba oil or sweet almond oil

- 10 drops chamomile essential oil

- 5 drops lavender essential oil

Instructions:

1. Mix oils together in a bottle.

2. Apply to damp skin after a shower.

Benefits: The carrier oil moisturizes, while chamomile and lavender soothe and relax the skin.

Body care is an essential part of self-care. By using natural ingredients, you not only nourish your skin but also ensure you're free from harmful chemicals often found in commercial products.

Embrace these recipes and enjoy the therapeutic process of creating and using them. Your skin will thank you!

CHAPTER 4: LIP AND ORAL CARE

A radiant smile can light up a room, and healthy lips can enhance that smile even further. This chapter is dedicated to the care of your lips and oral health, ensuring that your smile remains bright, and your lips stay soft and supple.

◆ ◆ ◆

4.1 Minty Lip Scrub

Ingredients:

- 1 tbsp sugar

- 1 tsp coconut oil

- 2 drops peppermint essential oil

Instructions:

1. Mix all ingredients in a small bowl.

2. Gently scrub onto lips in circular motions.

3. Rinse or wipe off.

Benefits: Sugar exfoliates, coconut oil moisturizes, and peppermint refreshes.

❖ ❖ ❖

4.2 Shea Butter Lip Balm

Ingredients:

- 2 tbsp shea butter

- 1 tbsp beeswax pellets

- 1 tbsp coconut oil

- 5 drops vanilla essential oil (optional)

Instructions:

1. In a double boiler, melt shea butter, beeswax, and coconut oil.

2. Once melted, remove from heat and add vanilla essential oil.

3. Pour into lip balm tubes or small tins. Allow to cool and solidify.

Benefits: Shea butter and coconut oil provide deep hydration, while beeswax seals in moisture.

❖ ❖ ❖

4.3 Natural Teeth Whitening Paste

Ingredients:

- 1 tbsp baking soda

- 1 tsp lemon juice

Instructions:

1. Mix baking soda and lemon juice to form a paste.

2. Apply to teeth using a toothbrush, brushing gently.

3. Leave for 2 minutes, then rinse thoroughly.

Benefits: Baking soda is a natural abrasive that can help remove surface stains, and lemon juice acts as a natural bleach.

❖ ❖ ❖

4.4 Herbal Mouthwash

Ingredients:

- 1 cup distilled water

- 2 tsp baking soda

- 5 drops tea tree essential oil

- 5 drops peppermint essential oil

Instructions:

1. Mix all ingredients in a bottle.

2. Shake well before each use. Swish in mouth for 30 seconds, then spit out.

Benefits: Baking soda neutralizes odors, tea tree oil has antibacterial properties, and peppermint oil freshens breath.

❖ ❖ ❖

4.5 Aloe Vera Lip Gel for Chapped Lips

Ingredients:

- 2 tbsp aloe vera gel

- 1 tsp honey

Instructions:

1. Mix aloe vera gel and honey in a small container.

2. Apply to chapped lips as needed.

Benefits: Aloe vera soothes and hydrates, while honey moisturizes and has antibacterial properties.

❖ ❖ ❖

4.6 Cinnamon Lip Plumper

Ingredients:

- 1 tbsp coconut oil

- 1 drop cinnamon essential oil

Instructions:

1. Mix coconut oil and cinnamon oil.

2. Apply a small amount to lips. You'll feel a tingling sensation.

3. Wipe off after 5 minutes.

Benefits: Cinnamon increases blood flow to the lips, making them appear fuller.

◆ ◆ ◆

4.7 Coconut Oil and Salt Tooth Scrub

Ingredients:

- 1 tbsp coconut oil

- 1 tsp sea salt

Instructions:

1. Mix coconut oil and sea salt.

2. Use as a toothpaste, brushing gently.

3. Rinse thoroughly.

Benefits: Coconut oil has antibacterial properties, and sea salt is a natural abrasive.

4.8 Berry Lip Tint

Ingredients:

- 1 tbsp coconut oil

- 1 tsp beeswax pellets

- 1 raspberry or blackberry (for color)

Instructions:

1. In a double boiler, melt coconut oil and beeswax.

2. Mash the berry and strain to get the juice. Add the juice to the melted mixture.

3. Pour into lip balm tubes or small tins. Allow to cool and solidify.

Benefits: Provides a natural tint while moisturizing the lips.

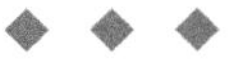

4.9 Clove Mouth Rinse for Toothache

Ingredients:

- 1 cup distilled water

- 5 drops clove essential oil

Instructions:

1. Mix water and clove oil in a bottle.

2. Swish in mouth for 30 seconds, focusing on the affected area, then spit out.

Benefits: Clove oil has natural analgesic and antibacterial properties, providing relief from toothache.

4.10 Honey and Vanilla Overnight Lip Mask

Ingredients:

- 1 tbsp honey

- 1 tbsp almond oil

- 5 drops vanilla essential oil

Instructions:

1. Mix all ingredients in a small container.

2. Apply a thick layer to lips before bed.

3. Wipe off in the morning.

Benefits: Deeply moisturizes and repairs lips while you sleep.

Oral and lip care is essential not just for aesthetic reasons but also for overall health. Using natural ingredients ensures that you're avoiding harmful chemicals while reaping the benefits of nature's bounty. Remember, a radiant smile and soft lips can be your best accessories!

CHAPTER 5: HAND AND FOOT CARE

Our hands and feet are among the most hardworking parts of our bodies. They endure daily stress, from walking and standing to typing and carrying. Despite their constant use, they often get the least amount of attention in our beauty routines. This chapter is dedicated to giving your hands and feet the care and pampering they deserve.

◆ ◆ ◆

5.1 Lemon and Sugar Hand Scrub

Ingredients:

- 2 tbsp sugar

- 1 tbsp olive oil

- 1 tsp lemon juice

Instructions:

1. Mix all ingredients in a bowl.

2. Gently scrub onto hands, focusing on knuckles and dry areas.

3. Rinse off with warm water.

Benefits: Sugar exfoliates dead skin cells, olive oil moisturizes, and lemon brightens.

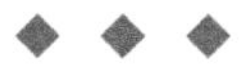

5.2 Eucalyptus Foot Soak

Ingredients:

- 1 cup Epsom salt

- 5 drops eucalyptus essential oil

- Warm water

Instructions:

1. Fill a basin with warm water.

2. Add Epsom salt and eucalyptus oil.

3. Soak feet for 15-20 minutes.

Benefits: Epsom salt relaxes tired feet, and eucalyptus provides a refreshing and antimicrobial touch.

5.3 Shea Butter Hand Cream

Ingredients:

- 1/2 cup shea butter

- 1/4 cup almond oil

- 10 drops lavender essential oil

Instructions:

1. In a double boiler, melt shea butter.

2. Once melted, mix in almond oil and lavender essential oil.

3. Pour into a jar and let set.

Benefits: Shea butter and almond oil deeply moisturize, while lavender soothes and adds a calming scent.

5.4 Peppermint Foot Cream

Ingredients:

- 1/2 cup coconut oil

- 1/4 cup beeswax pellets

- 10 drops peppermint essential oil

Instructions:

1. In a double boiler, melt coconut oil and beeswax.

2. Once melted, add peppermint essential oil.

3. Pour into a jar and let set.

Benefits: Coconut oil hydrates, beeswax forms a protective barrier, and peppermint refreshes tired feet.

5.5 Nail and Cuticle Oil

Ingredients:

- 1/4 cup jojoba oil

- 5 drops vitamin E oil

- 5 drops lavender essential oil

Instructions:

1. Mix all ingredients in a small bottle.

2. Apply to nails and cuticles, massaging gently.

Benefits: Jojoba oil and vitamin E nourish and strengthen nails, while lavender promotes healthy cuticles.

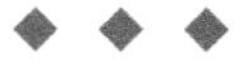

5.6 Oatmeal Hand Mask

Ingredients:

- 2 tbsp ground oatmeal

- 1 tbsp honey

- 1 tbsp yogurt

Instructions:

1. Mix all ingredients to form a paste.

2. Apply to hands, leaving on for 15 minutes.

3. Rinse off with warm water.

Benefits: Oatmeal soothes, honey moisturizes, and yogurt brightens the skin.

5.7 Clay Foot Mask for Detox

Ingredients:

- 1/2 cup bentonite clay

- 1/4 cup apple cider vinegar

- 5 drops tea tree essential oil

Instructions:

1. Mix clay and apple cider vinegar to form a paste.

2. Add tea tree oil and mix.

3. Apply to feet, leaving on for 20 minutes.

4. Rinse off with warm water.

Benefits: Bentonite clay draws out impurities, apple cider vinegar balances pH, and tea tree oil is antimicrobial.

5.8 Aloe Vera Hand Gel

Ingredients:

- 1/2 cup aloe vera gel

- 5 drops chamomile essential oil

Instructions:

1. Mix aloe vera gel and chamomile oil.

2. Apply to hands for instant hydration.

Benefits: Aloe vera hydrates and soothes, while chamomile reduces redness and irritation.

5.9 Pumice Foot Scrub

Ingredients:

- 2 tbsp ground pumice stone

- 1 tbsp coconut oil

- 5 drops lemon essential oil

Instructions:

1. Mix all ingredients to form a paste.

2. Scrub onto feet, focusing on heels and calloused areas.

3. Rinse off with warm water.

Benefits: Pumice exfoliates rough areas, coconut oil moisturizes, and lemon brightens.

5.10 Cooling Foot Spray

Ingredients:

- 1/2 cup witch hazel

- 1/4 cup distilled water

- 10 drops peppermint essential oil

Instructions:

1. Mix all ingredients in a spray bottle.

2. Spray onto feet for a refreshing and cooling sensation.

Benefits: Witch hazel tones and refreshes, while peppermint provides a cooling effect.

Your hands and feet are indicators of your overall health and well-being. By dedicating time to care for them, you not only enhance their appearance but also provide much-needed relaxation and rejuvenation. With these natural recipes, you can ensure they remain in top condition, ready to carry you through your daily tasks.

CHAPTER 6: EYE CARE

The eyes are often described as the windows to the soul. They express our emotions, convey our thoughts, and are essential for most of our daily tasks. However, the skin around the eyes is delicate and often shows the first signs of aging, fatigue, and stress. This chapter focuses on natural remedies and treatments to care for the eye area, ensuring it remains bright and youthful.

◆ ◆ ◆

6.1 Cucumber Eye Soothing Pads

Ingredients:

- Fresh cucumber slices

Instructions:

1. Refrigerate cucumber slices for 30 minutes.

2. Place the chilled slices over closed eyes.

3. Relax for 15-20 minutes, then remove.

Benefits: Cucumber has a cooling effect, reduces puffiness, and hydrates the skin.

◆ ◆ ◆

6.2 Aloe Vera Eye Gel for Puffiness

Ingredients:

- 2 tbsp aloe vera gel

- 5 drops chamomile essential oil

Instructions:

1. Mix aloe vera gel and chamomile oil.

2. Apply a small amount under the eyes.

3. Store the mixture in the refrigerator for added cooling.

Benefits: Aloe vera soothes and hydrates, while chamomile reduces inflammation and puffiness.

◆ ◆ ◆

6.3 Chamomile Eye Compress

Ingredients:

- 2 chamomile tea bags

- Warm water

Instructions:

1. Steep chamomile tea bags in warm water for 5 minutes.

2. Allow to cool slightly, then place the tea bags on closed eyes.

3. Relax for 15 minutes, then remove.

Benefits: Chamomile has anti-inflammatory properties that can help reduce redness and soothe tired eyes.

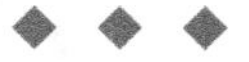

6.4 Coconut Oil Eye Cream

Ingredients:

- 2 tbsp coconut oil

- 5 drops vitamin E oil

- 3 drops lavender essential oil

Instructions:

1. Mix all ingredients until well combined.

2. Apply a small amount around the eyes before bedtime.

3. Store in a cool, dry place.

Benefits: Coconut oil moisturizes, vitamin E nourishes and repairs, and lavender soothes.

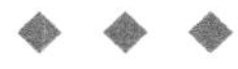

6.5 Green Tea Eye Pads for Dark Circles

Ingredients:

- 2 green tea bags

- Cold water

Instructions:

1. Steep green tea bags in cold water for 10 minutes.

2. Place the tea bags on closed eyes.

3. Relax for 20 minutes, then remove.

Benefits: Green tea contains antioxidants and caffeine that can help reduce dark circles and puffiness.

6.6 Rosehip Oil Serum for Fine Lines

Ingredients:

- 2 tbsp rosehip oil

- 5 drops frankincense essential oil

Instructions:

1. Mix rosehip oil and frankincense oil.

2. Apply a few drops around the eyes, gently patting with fingertips.

3. Use nightly.

Benefits: Rosehip oil promotes skin regeneration and reduces signs of aging, while frankincense can help tighten and firm the skin.

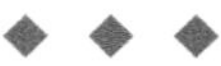

6.7 Potato Slice Treatment for Dark Circles

Ingredients:

- Fresh potato slices

Instructions:

1. Refrigerate potato slices for 30 minutes.

2. Place the chilled slices over closed eyes.

3. Relax for 15-20 minutes, then remove.

Benefits: Potatoes contain enzymes that can help lighten dark circles and reduce puffiness.

6.8 Avocado Eye Mask

Ingredients:

- 1/4 ripe avocado

- 1 tsp almond oil

Instructions:

1. Mash avocado and mix with almond oil.

2. Apply the mixture under the eyes.

3. Leave on for 10-15 minutes, then rinse.

Benefits: Avocado hydrates and nourishes the skin, while almond oil provides added moisture and reduces the appearance of fine lines.

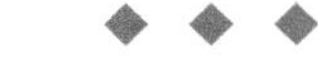

6.9 Carrot Seed Eye Serum

Ingredients:
- 2 tbsp jojoba oil
- 5 drops carrot seed essential oil

Instructions:

1. Mix jojoba oil and carrot seed oil.

2. Apply a few drops around the eyes, gently patting with fingertips.

3. Use nightly.

Benefits: Carrot seed oil rejuvenates and revitalizes the skin, helping to smooth fine lines and wrinkles.

6.10 DIY Eye Makeup Remover

Ingredients:
- 2 tbsp witch hazel
- 2 tbsp olive oil or jojoba oil

Instructions:

1. Mix witch hazel and oil in a bottle.

2. Shake well before each use.

3. Apply to a cotton pad and gently wipe away eye makeup.

Benefits: The oil breaks down makeup, while witch hazel soothes and cleanses the skin.

Eye care is a crucial aspect of a holistic beauty routine. The skin around the eyes is sensitive and requires gentle, yet effective treatments. By incorporating these natural remedies, you can address common eye concerns and ensure that your eyes remain bright, youthful, and expressive.

CHAPTER 7: NATURAL PERFUMES AND DEODORANTS

Scent has the power to evoke memories, influence moods, and define personalities. While commercial perfumes and deodorants can be filled with chemicals and synthetic fragrances, natural alternatives offer a refreshing and skin-friendly approach. This chapter delves into crafting personal scents and effective deodorants using nature's bounty.

◆ ◆ ◆

7.1 Basic Solid Perfume

Ingredients:

- 2 tbsp jojoba oil or sweet almond oil

- 1 tbsp beeswax pellets

- 15-20 drops of your favorite essential oil or blend

Instructions:

1. In a double boiler, melt beeswax and oil together.

2. Remove from heat and let cool slightly.

3. Add essential oils and mix well.

4. Pour into small tins or containers and let set.

Benefits: A customizable scent that's easy to carry and apply.

7.2 Lavender and Rose Roll-On Perfume

Ingredients:

- 2 tbsp jojoba oil

- 10 drops lavender essential oil

- 5 drops rose essential oil

Instructions:

1. In a roll-on bottle, add the essential oils.

2. Fill the rest of the bottle with jojoba oil.

3. Cap and shake well before each use.

Benefits: A calming and romantic scent in a convenient roll-on format.

7.3 Baking Soda-Free Natural Deodorant

Ingredients:

- 3 tbsp coconut oil

- 2 tbsp arrowroot powder or cornstarch

- 2 tbsp shea butter

- 10 drops tea tree essential oil

Instructions:

1. In a double boiler, melt coconut oil and shea butter.

2. Remove from heat and whisk in arrowroot powder or cornstarch.

3. Add tea tree oil and mix well.

4. Pour into an empty deodorant container or a small jar. Allow to solidify.

Benefits: Effective odor protection without the potential irritation of baking soda.

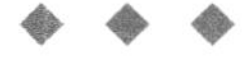

7.4 Citrus Spray Deodorant

Ingredients:
- 1/2 cup witch hazel
- 1/4 cup aloe vera gel
- 10 drops lemon essential oil
- 10 drops bergamot essential oil

Instructions:
1. Mix all ingredients in a spray bottle.
2. Shake well before each use. Spray underarms as needed.

Benefits: A refreshing and uplifting scent that neutralizes odors.

7.5 Floral Solid Perfume

Ingredients:
- 2 tbsp jojoba oil
- 1 tbsp beeswax pellets
- 7 drops jasmine essential oil

- 7 drops ylang-ylang essential oil

- 6 drops rose essential oil

Instructions:

1. In a double boiler, melt beeswax and jojoba oil.

2. Remove from heat and add essential oils.

3. Pour into a small tin or locket. Allow to solidify.

Benefits: A rich and luxurious floral scent.

7.6 Herbal Deodorant Stick

Ingredients:

- 3 tbsp coconut oil

- 2 tbsp baking soda

- 2 tbsp arrowroot powder

- 2 tbsp beeswax pellets

- 10 drops lavender essential oil

- 5 drops rosemary essential oil

Instructions:

1. Melt beeswax, coconut oil in a double boiler.

2. Remove from heat and mix in baking soda and arrowroot powder.

3. Add essential oils and stir.

4. Pour into empty deodorant containers. Allow to solidify.

Benefits: Long-lasting protection with a calming herbal scent.

7.7 Vanilla and Sandalwood Perfume Oil

Ingredients:

- 2 tbsp jojoba oil

- 10 drops vanilla absolute

- 10 drops sandalwood essential oil

Instructions:

1. In a small bottle, mix jojoba oil with essential oils.

2. Roll between palms to mix. Apply to pulse points as desired.

Benefits: A warm and sensual scent.

7.8 Charcoal and Tea Tree Deodorant Cream

Ingredients:

- 3 tbsp coconut oil

- 1 tbsp activated charcoal powder

- 2 tbsp arrowroot powder

- 10 drops tea tree essential oil

Instructions:

1. Mix coconut oil, activated charcoal, and arrowroot powder to form a paste.

2. Add tea tree oil and mix well.

3. Store in a small jar. Apply a pea-sized amount to underarms with fingers.

Benefits: Activated charcoal helps neutralize odors, and tea tree offers antimicrobial properties.

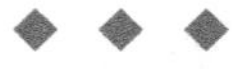

7.9 Herbal Deodorant Powder

Ingredients:

1/4 cup arrowroot powder

1 tbsp baking soda

5 drops lavender essential oil

5 drops tea tree essential oil

Instructions:

Mix all ingredients in a jar.

Apply a small amount to underarms using a makeup brush or puff.

Benefits: Arrowroot and baking soda absorb moisture, while lavender and tea tree provide a pleasant scent and antibacterial properties.

7.10 Sandalwood and Vanilla Body Mist

Ingredients:

1/2 cup distilled water

10 drops sandalwood essential oil

5 drops vanilla absolute

Instructions:

Mix all ingredients in a spray bottle.

Shake well before each use. Mist over body for a warm, comforting scent.

Benefits: Sandalwood provides a deep, woody base, while vanilla adds a sweet, comforting top note.

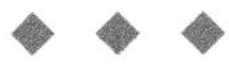

7.11 Probiotic Deodorant Cream

Ingredients:

3 tbsp coconut oil

1 tbsp beeswax pellets

2 tbsp arrowroot powder

1 capsule probiotic (powder)

10 drops lavender essential oil

Instructions:

In a double boiler, melt coconut oil and beeswax.

Remove from heat and mix in arrowroot powder.

Open the probiotic capsule and mix the powder into the mixture.

Add lavender essential oil and stir.

Store in a small jar. Apply a pea-sized amount to underarms with fingers.

Benefits: Probiotics help balance skin's natural flora, reducing odor-causing bacteria. Lavender adds a calming scent.

Natural perfumes and deodorants not only provide the desired effects of scent and freshness but also ensure that you're free from harmful chemicals often found in commercial products. Crafting your own scents and deodorants allows for personalization and the peace of mind that comes from knowing exactly what's touching your skin. Embrace the art of natural fragrance and feel confident in your choices.

50

CHAPTER 8: HOLISTIC WELLNESS AND STRESS RELIEF

Holistic wellness goes beyond mere physical health. It encompasses mental, emotional, and spiritual well-being. In our fast-paced lives, stress can take a toll on all these aspects. This chapter focuses on natural remedies and practices that promote overall wellness and provide relief from stress and anxiety.

8.1 Lavender Stress Relief Bath Soak

Ingredients:

- 1 cup Epsom salt

- 1/2 cup baking soda

- 10 drops lavender essential oil

Instructions:

1. Mix all ingredients in a bowl.

2. Add to a warm bath and soak for 20-30 minutes.

Benefits: Epsom salt relaxes muscles, baking soda softens skin, and lavender calms the mind.

8.2 Peppermint Headache Relief Roller

Ingredients:

- 10 drops peppermint essential oil

- 2 tbsp carrier oil (such as jojoba or almond oil)

Instructions:

1. Mix peppermint oil with the carrier oil in a roll-on bottle.

2. Apply to temples and back of the neck as needed for headache relief.

Benefits: Peppermint oil can reduce headache symptoms through its cooling and calming effects.

8.3 Chamomile Sleep Aid Tea

Ingredients:

- 1 tbsp dried chamomile flowers

- 1 cup hot water

Instructions:

1. Steep chamomile flowers in hot water for 5-7 minutes.

2. Strain and enjoy before bedtime.

Benefits: Chamomile has natural calming properties that can aid in relaxation and sleep.

$$\diamond \quad \diamond \quad \diamond$$

8.4 Yoga and Meditation Practice

Instructions:

1. Find a quiet space and comfortable position.

2. Focus on deep breathing, inhaling and exhaling slowly.

3. Incorporate gentle yoga stretches or meditation techniques.

4. Practice regularly for best results.

Benefits: Yoga and meditation can reduce stress, improve mental clarity, and enhance overall well-being.

$$\diamond \quad \diamond \quad \diamond$$

8.5 Rosemary Memory Boost Inhaler

Ingredients:

- 10 drops rosemary essential oil
- Inhaler stick

Instructions:

1. Add rosemary essential oil to the inhaler stick.

2. Inhale deeply whenever you need a mental boost.

Benefits: Rosemary is known to enhance memory and concentration.

$$\diamond \quad \diamond \quad \diamond$$

8.6 Ginger and Lemon Immunity Tea

Ingredients:

- 1-inch fresh ginger, sliced
- 1 lemon, sliced

- 1 tbsp honey

- 2 cups hot water

Instructions:

1. Add ginger and lemon to hot water.

2. Steep for 10 minutes, then add honey.

3. Enjoy warm to support immune health.

Benefits: Ginger and lemon provide vitamin C and antioxidants, while honey adds soothing properties.

8.7 Frankincense Mood Lifting Diffuser Blend

Ingredients:

- 5 drops frankincense essential oil

- 5 drops orange essential oil

- Diffuser

Instructions:

1. Add essential oils to a diffuser.

2. Enjoy the uplifting aroma throughout the day.

Benefits: Frankincense and orange essential oils can elevate mood and reduce feelings of depression.

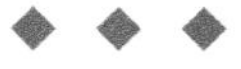

8.8 DIY Massage Oil for Muscle Relaxation

Ingredients:

- 1 cup almond oil

- 10 drops lavender essential oil

- 5 drops eucalyptus essential oil

Instructions:

1. Mix all ingredients in a bottle.

2. Use for self-massage or have a partner massage tense areas.

Benefits: Almond oil nourishes the skin, while lavender and eucalyptus relax muscles.

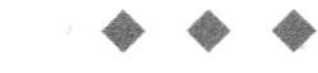

8.9 Herbal Pillow Spray for Restful Sleep

Ingredients:

- 1/2 cup distilled water

- 10 drops lavender essential oil

- 5 drops chamomile essential oil

Instructions:

1. Mix all ingredients in a spray bottle.

2. Mist over pillows and linens before bedtime.

Benefits: Lavender and chamomile promote relaxation and aid in restful sleep.

8.10 Journaling for Emotional Well-being

Instructions:

1. Find a quiet space and a journal or notebook.

2. Write down thoughts, feelings, and reflections.

3. Make it a regular practice, especially during stressful times.

Benefits: Journaling can provide emotional release, enhance self-awareness, and support mental health.

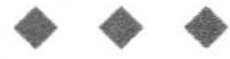

Holistic wellness recognizes the interconnectedness of body, mind, and spirit. By incorporating natural remedies and mindful practices, you can create a balanced and harmonious life. Whether it's through herbal teas, essential oils, or mindful exercises, these methods offer a gentle way to nurture yourself and cope with life's challenges. Remember, self-care is not a luxury; it's a necessity for overall well-being.

CHAPTER 9: MEN'S CARE

While the beauty and wellness industry has historically been geared towards women, the importance of specialized care for men cannot be understated. Men's skin and hair have unique needs, influenced by factors like facial hair, hormones, and often different daily routines. This chapter offers a collection of homemade recipes tailored for the modern man, ensuring that he too can enjoy the benefits of natural care.

9.1 Beard Oil for Softness and Shine

Ingredients:

- 2 tbsp jojoba oil

- 1 tbsp argan oil

- 5 drops cedarwood essential oil

- 3 drops tea tree essential oil

Instructions:

1. Mix all ingredients in a small bottle.

2. Apply a few drops to the beard, massaging it in to nourish both the hair and the skin underneath.

Benefits: Softens beard hair, adds shine, and has antiseptic properties.

9.2 Natural Aftershave Lotion

Ingredients:

- 1/2 cup witch hazel

- 1/4 cup aloe vera gel

- 5 drops lavender essential oil

- 3 drops chamomile essential oil

Instructions:

1. Combine all ingredients in a bottle and shake well.

2. Apply to freshly shaved skin to soothe and prevent irritation.

Benefits: Reduces redness, soothes razor burns, and hydrates the skin.

9.3 Hair Pomade for Styling

Ingredients:

- 2 tbsp shea butter

- 1 tbsp beeswax pellets

- 2 tbsp coconut oil

- 5 drops sandalwood essential oil

Instructions:

1. Melt shea butter, beeswax, and coconut oil in a double boiler.

2. Remove from heat and stir in sandalwood essential oil.

3. Pour into a small jar and allow to solidify.

4. Use a small amount to style hair as desired.

Benefits: Provides hold for styling, moisturizes hair, and offers a pleasant scent.

9.4 Exfoliating Face Scrub

Ingredients:

- 1/2 cup ground coffee

- 1/4 cup brown sugar

- 1/4 cup coconut oil

Instructions:

1. Mix all ingredients to form a paste.

2. Gently massage onto wet face in circular motions.

3. Rinse with warm water.

Benefits: Exfoliates dead skin cells, invigorates the skin, and moisturizes.

9.5 Natural Deodorant for Men

Ingredients:

- 2 tbsp coconut oil

- 2 tbsp baking soda

- 2 tbsp arrowroot powder

- 5 drops eucalyptus essential oil

- 5 drops pine essential oil

Instructions:

1. Mix all ingredients to form a paste.

2. Store in a small jar.

3. Apply a small amount to underarms daily.

Benefits: Neutralizes odor, absorbs moisture, and provides a fresh, masculine scent.

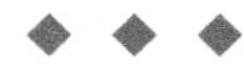

9.6 Moisturizing Hand Salve

Ingredients:

- 1/4 cup shea butter

- 1/8 cup beeswax pellets

- 1/4 cup almond oil

- 5 drops frankincense essential oil

Instructions:

1. Melt shea butter, beeswax, and almond oil in a double boiler.

2. Remove from heat and add frankincense essential oil.

3. Pour into a small tin or jar and allow to solidify.

Benefits: Deeply moisturizes, heals cracked skin, and soothes.

9.7 Foot Soak for Tired Feet

Ingredients:

- 1 cup Epsom salt

- 1/2 cup sea salt

- 5 drops peppermint essential oil

- Warm water

Instructions:

1. Fill a basin with warm water.

2. Add Epsom salt, sea salt, and peppermint essential oil.

3. Soak feet for 15-20 minutes.

Benefits: Relaxes tired muscles, detoxifies, and refreshes.

9.8 Invigorating Body Wash

Ingredients:

- 1/2 cup unscented castile soap

- 1/4 cup honey

- 1/4 cup coconut oil (melted)

- 10 drops rosemary essential oil

- 7 drops bergamot essential oil

Instructions:

1. In a mixing bowl, combine the castile soap, honey, and melted coconut oil.

2. Stir until well combined.

3. Add the essential oils and mix thoroughly.

4. Transfer to a squeeze or pump bottle.

5. Use as you would any regular body wash during showers.

Benefits: Cleanses the skin without stripping natural oils, invigorates the senses, and provides moisture.

9.9 Energizing Hair Tonic

Ingredients:

- 1 cup distilled water

- 2 tbsp apple cider vinegar

- 5 drops cedarwood essential oil

- 5 drops peppermint essential oil

Instructions:

1. Combine all ingredients in a spray bottle.

2. After shampooing, spray the tonic onto the scalp and massage gently.

3. Rinse with cool water or leave in for a refreshing sensation.

Benefits: Stimulates the scalp, promotes hair growth, and balances pH levels.

9.10 Overnight Hydrating Face Mask

Ingredients:

- 2 tbsp aloe vera gel

- 1 tbsp almond oil

- 5 drops lavender essential oil

- 3 drops vitamin E oil

Instructions:

1. In a small bowl, mix the aloe vera gel and almond oil.

2. Add the essential oil and vitamin E oil, mixing thoroughly.

3. Apply a thin layer to the face before bedtime.

4. Rinse off in the morning with lukewarm water.

Benefits: Deeply hydrates the skin, reduces inflammation, and promotes skin healing and rejuvenation.

With these additional recipes, men can further enhance their self-care routine, ensuring that from head to toe, they are using products that not only improve their appearance but also promote overall skin and hair health. Whether it's the invigorating sensation of an energizing body wash or the deep hydration of an overnight mask, these recipes cater to the diverse needs of men's skin and hair care.

CHAPTER 10: MISCELLANEOUS

This chapter explores a diverse range of recipes that don't fit into traditional categories but offer unique and valuable additions to your natural beauty and wellness routine.

◆ ◆ ◆

10.1 DIY Natural Toothpaste

Ingredients:

- 2 tbsp coconut oil

- 1 tbsp baking soda

- 10 drops peppermint essential oil

Instructions:

1. Mix all ingredients to form a paste.

2. Store in a small jar and use as regular toothpaste.

Benefits: A fluoride-free alternative that cleans teeth and freshens breath.

◆ ◆ ◆

10.2 Homemade Fabric Freshener Spray

Ingredients:

- 1 cup distilled water

- 1/4 cup vodka or rubbing alcohol

- 10 drops lavender essential oil

Instructions:

1. Mix all ingredients in a spray bottle.

2. Spray on fabrics to refresh and deodorize.

Benefits: A natural way to freshen fabrics without synthetic fragrances.

◆ ◆ ◆

10.3 Natural Insect Repellent Lotion

Ingredients:

- 1/2 cup shea butter

- 1/4 cup coconut oil

- 10 drops citronella essential oil

- 10 drops eucalyptus essential oil

Instructions:

1. Melt shea butter and coconut oil in a double boiler.

2. Remove from heat and add essential oils.

3. Pour into a jar and allow to solidify.

Benefits: A skin-friendly insect repellent without harsh chemicals.

◆ ◆ ◆

10.4 Herbal Sleep Aid Tea

Ingredients:

- 1 tbsp dried chamomile flowers

- 1 tbsp dried lavender flowers

- 1 tsp dried lemon balm

Instructions:

1. Mix herbs and steep in hot water for 5-7 minutes.

2. Strain and enjoy before bedtime.

Benefits: A calming tea blend to promote restful sleep.

❖ ❖ ❖

10.5 DIY Silk Hair Serum

Ingredients:

- 2 tbsp jojoba oil

- 5 drops silk amino acids

- 5 drops rosemary essential oil

Instructions:

1. Mix all ingredients in a small bottle.

2. Apply a few drops to damp or dry hair to smooth and shine.

Benefits: A nourishing serum that mimics the benefits of silk for hair.

❖ ❖ ❖

10.6 Epsom Salt Foot Soak

Ingredients:

- 1 cup Epsom salt

- 5 drops tea tree essential oil

- Warm water

Instructions:

1. Fill a basin with warm water and add Epsom salt and tea tree oil.

2. Soak feet for 15-20 minutes.

Benefits: A relaxing foot soak that softens skin and fights fungal infections.

◆ ◆ ◆

10.7 Natural Air Purifying Spray

Ingredients:

- 1 cup distilled water

- 10 drops lemon essential oil

- 10 drops pine essential oil

Instructions:

1. Mix all ingredients in a spray bottle.

2. Mist around the home to purify the air.

Benefits: A fresh and natural way to cleanse the air without artificial fragrances.

◆ ◆ ◆

10.8 DIY Stress-Relief Bath Salts

Ingredients:

- 1 cup Epsom salt

- 1/2 cup sea salt

- 10 drops lavender essential oil

- 5 drops chamomile essential oil

Instructions:

1. Mix all ingredients and store in a jar.

2. Add a handful to a warm bath and soak.

Benefits: A calming bath soak to relieve stress and soothe muscles.

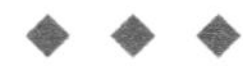

10.9 Homemade Lip Balm with Honey

Ingredients:

- 2 tbsp beeswax pellets

- 2 tbsp coconut oil

- 1 tsp honey

Instructions:

1. Melt beeswax and coconut oil in a double boiler.

2. Remove from heat and stir in honey.

3. Pour into lip balm tubes or small containers.

Benefits: A nourishing lip balm that hydrates and protects.

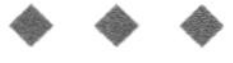

10.10 Natural Yoga Mat Cleaner

Ingredients:

- 1 cup distilled water

- 1/4 cup witch hazel

- 10 drops tea tree essential oil

- 5 drops lavender essential oil

Instructions:

1. Mix all ingredients in a spray bottle.

2. Spray on the yoga mat and wipe clean.

Benefits: A gentle cleaner that disinfects without damaging the mat.

This chapter's miscellaneous recipes offer a wide array of natural solutions for everyday needs. From personal care to home freshness, these recipes allow you to embrace a holistic lifestyle that aligns with nature. Experimenting with these diverse recipes can lead to delightful discoveries and enhance your overall well-being.